NOT EVERYTHING IS BLACK & WHITE

BY

L.W.
CARRINSON

Cover design by: L.W. CARRINSON

Publisher: L.W. CARRINSON

Copyright enquiries: lwcarrinson@gmail.com

Contents

INTRODUCTION

I'm just going to explain to you the title on the front of this book and what it represents to me and why I chose it.

For me it is the contrast as to how I see life and what I call "normal" people see life. Normal people see life in black and white but also understand the grey in the middle, they have the ability to weigh everything up and make decisions in their lives, but from my own personal point of view and living with depression, anxiety and EUPD (emotionally unstable personality disorder), I see life in just black and white, sadly there is no in-between or weighing things up for me, there is no grey, as some of my poems express.

You will read about my story and some of the dark places I have experienced.

The dark face represents me (or maybe yourself) going through a really dark time but masking my way through life with that 'everything is ok fake smile.'

The light face represents light at the end of the tunnel and things around me can be really good at times but the fake mask can't hide the sadness and pain that was going on inside me but there was light, there was hope and I found the courage to get through the bad times.

Hope you enjoy reading my poems and reading the reasons behind each poem. I hope you realise that you're not alone even though you're going through your loneliest journey, and that there is a way forward and the grey will appear at points in your life you least expect them to.

NANNY BRENDA

My Nan was special, my Nan was the best,
Now she is in heaven, so I'll let her rest,

She always put us first and never let us down,
She always gave a smile but never gave a frown,

She loved her family and she loved her home,
She was always there when we needed to moan,

She leaves a big hole but nothing to say,
Why did it have to be this way,

You were special in every way,
But now there is nothing left to say.

Nan Brenda

NANNY BRENDA EXPLANATION

I was born in 1985 and was only 12 years old when my Nan died and this was the first poem I had ever written. She was a lovely lady my Nan, but I don't really remember much from my past, not sure if that's because I blocked a lot of things out from the events that were about to unfold in my life or if I simply had so much that had happened, my brain can't process it all.

Anyway, there are three things that stand out about my Nan.

The first thing I remember was her laugh, she would always sit with her hands underneath the tops of her legs not really sure why she did, but I always remember her doing it while sitting in her front room, she would be chatting away, (hands under her legs) then something funny was said and that was it, her infectious loud laugh filled the room, I swear she nearly peed herself a few times because she laughed so hard and so long like she was never going to stop.

The second thing that stands out about my nan was one particular Christmas time, it was always so busy at my nans, well she did have seven children so you can imagine all my aunts and uncles and their partners and kids were all there. One uncle in particular was trying to show my Nan a card game, (She didn't really understand card games), But my uncle asked my Nan if she knew how to play '52 card pick up', my Nan not having a clue, obviously replied no, so my uncle started shuffling all the cards all professional like then he just threw all the cards on the floor and

then said to my Nan "now you have to pick them all up", we all started laughing and I think we laughed for hours after that and it's something I will never forget.

The third thing I remember about my Nan was her cooking, she was always a good cook, both my Nans were actually, maybe that's just a Nan thing I don't really know but she did make the best dinners.

I know to this day that my mum would eat my Nans Yorkshire puddings because she made the best ones ever. When my nan passed away my mum hasn't eaten a Yorkshire pudding since, there isn't one that could match up to my Nans for her.

HIT OF THE YEAR

I was growing up and fell in love when I was very young,
But the hell I was about to experience had only just begun,

I met a 'boy', who I thought I'd be with for the rest of my life,
Things were going ok; we got engaged and later thought I'd be his wife,

But then I fell pregnant with our beautiful baby girl,
But I was too blind to see I was about to go through hell,

The arguments started because my emotions were changing,
And I knew bit by bit my heart was breaking,

All this changed and everything seemed to fall in place,
But he wasn't ready to be a father, that's when I got my first smack in the face,

The arguments got bad so I went my own way,
But his words made me miss him every single day,

So, we got back together and things were going great,
But it was a matter of days before it all turned to hate,

My Mum moved away and I felt all on my own,
But all I could do was cry down the phone,

Being hit all the time was a part of my life... But I didn't know why,
I smiled and put on a brave face when all I wanted to do was cry,

Things all came to an end when I couldn't take no more,
He hit me again so I walked out the door.

HIT OF THE YEAR EXPLANATION

I met 'him' when I was around 17, seemed like a nice boy (at that time). That was until his true colours started coming through.

It started with small things from him like commenting on my tops being 'too low' or asking what I had spent all my money on (to the point I added up every single penny in case he thought I had spent it on...), well God only knows, but me being naive at 17, I thought it was normal, I didn't know any different.

'Him' and drink did not mix at all, that's when I got my first slap, obviously he apologised the next day and it was never going to happen again.

By this time, our baby girl was born. We had only been together 3 months before I fell pregnant, she was with the babysitter on one of the nights I got smacked AGAIN.

On this night we had been down the pub, he was smiling and laughing and joking and I could see that everyone in there thought he was the doting dad, perfect partner and just an all-round top guy. Yeah, that was until we got home.

He carried on drinking, as he always did and I can still remember what it was he was drinking and the awful strong smell of it. It was Jack Daniel's and Coke. I hate any whiskey and the smell of it makes me feel sick. I'm not sure if I genuinely don't like the smell of it or because of the memories it brings back.

Then bang... in a split second I couldn't breathe, his hands were tightly gripped around my throat and I couldn't get any air to my lungs, I was trying so hard to shout but nothing came out, the feeling of not being able to breath will stay with me for as long as I live.

Then slowly I felt his grip loosen from my throat and I could feel my lungs starting to fill with air again, thank God for that.

Then BANG again in a split second he punched me straight in the eye and that instantly took away the feeling of not being able to breath just moments before.

I held my eye thinking 'what the F did I say', 'what did I do', 'who did I speak to', but nothing came to me, just the swelling and my tears stinging my already bruised and swollen eye.

Then came his tears, yes, HIS tears. Why did he deserve to be crying, it was me that was hurt, me that couldn't breathe for them few seconds (that felt like minutes,) yet HE was crying, crying like our baby would, he just kept saying sorry over and over and that it would never happen again, (which it did so much I lost count, this is just a few I've included in this book).

He said sorry so many times I even started to feel sorry for him and not in a pity way like genuinely sorry for him.

In the morning I remember him looking over at me with this shocked look on his face, that's when I thought, God my eye must look even worse this morning, but nope, he had no idea what he had done to me, he then asked if we got into a fight at the pub.

I thought 'really', I was so angry at that point; I told him exactly what had happened and what he had done to me and yet again, I heard that familiar word, 'sorry' but let's face it how can someone be truly sorry for something they have no knowledge of doing?

Slowly over the days my eye went down, he even brought me some witch-hazel to help, (Generous of him I know).

Once my eye was nearly healed, (well to the point my make-up covered it), I started going out again and seeing family (which he didn't really like anyway).

It wasn't long after my daughter was born that my Mum moved away, I actually didn't realise how much I needed her, but of course I couldn't say why, as far as she was aware I was happy and had a wonderful partner and gorgeous little family, but I actually wanted her to come and protect me from all the abuse I still had to come.

I left him after about a year, but I always ended up back in the same situation because I was weak and brain washed and lost all confidence in myself. I suppose I just wanted to be loved by the father of my child, but I couldn't unless that involved all the hurt along the way, he made sure I knew, (at the time), that no other man would or could love me, only him, because I was too disgusting for anyone else.

So, there I was being hit, accepting his apologies and trying to believe his endless promises.

HE

He slapped me, he punched me,
He kicked me he bit me,

He got in my head with his twisted brain,
He made me feel like I was going insane,

He tied me up he ripped my clothes,
He loved the colours blue and mauve,

He always said sorry then came his tears,
He made me live in complete an utter fear,

He punched me hard while holding my boy,
He hurt me bad like I was just a toy,

He controlled my brain an everyday life,
He actually asked me to be his wife,

He made me stay in to cover up my face,
He made me think I was a total disgrace,

He beat me in the street, he jumped on my back,
He kicked me in the ribs with his steel toe caps,

He strangled me so hard I went totally blue,
He lied so much that no one had a clue,

He lied to the police so I had too as well,
He made sure of that or there would be hell,

He made me take him back all over again,
He made me believe that this was just men,

He made me fight back after years of hurt,
He made everyone think it was me that was dirt,

He made people see it wasn't just him,
He made people see it was me that would win,

He made me out to be shallow and low,
He made people believe I gave the last blow,

He made me fight back for the sake of my kids,
He made me believe what I did was sick,

But was I wrong to defend myself,
For the sake of my babies and my mental health?

HE EXPLANATION

The years had gone by and I was trapped, trapped in this vicious circle of hit, hurt, cry, apologies and start all over again. It was never ending and I thought at this point this was my life, either until I lost my mind and done something stupid or he killed me, that was the only two options I felt I was left with.

We ended up getting a house just round the corner from his Mum, another fresh start that I knew deep down would never last. on this particular day my baby girl was with her Nan just round the corner from us and yet again an argument had happened, he as usual was stoned and drunk.

I can still remember what I was wearing, crazy how I remember irrelevant details. Anyway, I had cream coloured loose three quartered length trousers on, with a white top and a little angel broach my mum had sent me from Australia, made me feel like an angel was watching over me, (how wrong was I), the next few hours of my life were another little piece of hell for me.

I must have been giving him some mouth, because at that point I knew I couldn't fight back, but the one thing I did have, was my evil tongue. To me that was my way of fighting back, it was my weapon to make me feel like I had at least done something to hurt him, even if it was with words.

I wanted him to feel some sort of pain, pain he had done to me with his hands and if that meant I had to use my tongue, then so be it.

I must have really pushed his buttons this time though and said something that hit a nerve, because he put his hands around my throat AGAIN and pushed me so far back that I was arched over the baby's cot backwards, and again not being able to breath.

He had been at work earlier that morning so had his steel toe cap boots on, and after dragging and pulling me around the room by my hair, I felt one of them boots kick me straight in the leg, he kicked me so hard I had the print of his boot on my trouser leg and when I saw later on it was imprinted on the outside of my skin too.

The police to this day, still have these clothes, as I refused to collect them, (why would I?)

I remember curling up in a ball to protect my face, then the next thing I know, I'm being dragged down the stairs by my hair, he then pulled a chair from our dining room table and dragged it behind him with his spare hand to the living room, there he shoved me down to sit on it like I was a prisoner.

He then tied my hands behind me with black electrical tape.

He hit me a few times while threatening to do worse things to me and he was just rambling on and on about things that didn't even make sense. He then poured a bottle of coke all over me.

This made me feel worthless in every way possible, not sure why but it just felt degrading.

I remember being angrier at the fact the coke splashes had gone on a painting that my dad had made for me which was of my Mum and I.

I don't know how long I was tied up (felt like hours) but then he must have calmed down because he cut the tape off my hands and this is when my anger kicked in because I no longer felt powerless.

I was saying all sorts to him and shouting at him for everything he had done to me, but then he just reached for me and threw me on the floor like a ragdoll and ripped my white top open so my bra could be seen. This is where I thought he was going to rape me (he threatened too) but he didn't.

I don't really remember much after that because he hit me a few more times and most of it was a blur.

I do remember him going to the toilet, and that's when I knew I had to get out of there, so I ran to the front door, unlocked it and ran as fast as I could round the corner to his Mum's house with my top ripped open, blood pouring down my face, covered in coke and barefooted, I ran until I got to her door and knocked as quickly and loudly as I could.

She opened the door and I ran past her inside to make me feel a bit safer. Then the police were called and he was arrested (one time of many to come). The police took all my wet blooded clothes as evidence.

The next day he was out again, I felt deflated like why did I bother, I was getting nowhere and I was stuck in this dark circle and I was tired of going round and round in it, I just wanted some peace, I was tired physically and mentally and didn't know how long I could carry on doing the same thing, how do I escape this?

ONE MORE

Let's have a drink, vodka or wine,
Mind you any drink will do as long as it's mine,

The more I drink the happier I get,
Just one more and I know I'll forget,

Forget the last blow that I've just had to take,
Be the happy girl without them knowing I'm fake,

Dance about like I'm having a blast,
He told me that punch would be the last,

He lied again so now I need a drink,
The more I have the quicker I sink,

I didn't want the drinking to ever stop,
But it will do soon then I'll just drop,

I'll wake the next day and there I'll see,
Another black eye staring back at me,

I'll open a bottle and have just one more,
I don't really know if I can take anymore.

ONE MORE EXPLANATION

Drink became a big part of my life for quite some time. At the time I thought it was great, I felt confident, I felt like I could take on the world, I thought I forgot about the arguments, fights and name calling, I danced around like I was on this high that no one could bring me down from.

But it was still there, the thoughts, the feelings, the wondering of what was next for me.

The drink just made it easier for me to cope with and on the plus side it didn't hurt as much when he hit, bit, kicked or punched me.

It started off as some low percent wine that I was necking daily. the more I drank the more my body felt like it was floating, I felt like I could mask my smiles. It made me not care about what was going to happen, then it turned to stronger wine, the low percent just wasn't cutting it anymore.

It made me sleep, which I felt like I hadn't slept properly in years. Always sleeping with 'One eye open' as they say because I never knew what the unpredictable 'boy' had in mind for me next.

I would wake some mornings after yet another argument that turned physical and go straight to the bathroom as you do and there it was, another black eye, or bruised cheek or fat lip. Again, on the plus side I didn't feel it (at the time) but I sure did right then, standing there looking in the mirror, my numbing friend (drink) was slowly leaving my body so I felt the bruises or cuts or soreness that was staring back at me.

Best thing to do was pour open the wine and forget it ever happened AGAIN.

It was taking too long for the wine to kick in this time so I went onto the vodka, worst thing I could have ever drunk, that sent me to a whole new level. It made me want to dance round the room like life was amazing for me but it was all a cover up, I knew that deep down anyway, I just became good at pretending and masking my hurt and pain.

The mornings after were the worst for me because the drink had worn off and I was left with the most depressing, suicidal thoughts I could have had. Obviously, drink is a depressant anyway and the way I felt each morning before a drink was the worst. I didn't want to be alive; I didn't want to keep living in this same circle of hell but getting out of it didn't seem like an option at the time.

So off I went downstairs to find the alcohol and I went on like this for a long time until something clicked in my head, it was looking at my children. I had to be strong for them because they were also living this nightmare but they couldn't drown their feelings out, they couldn't fight back and they certainly didn't deserve to have an alcoholic as a mum. I was the mum, I had to protect them no matter what and that meant putting or rather blocking my thoughts and feelings out for them, I had no idea by doing this it would then turn to the many problems I had later in life.

It all catches up with you in the end, the past affects the present and sometimes the future but it's how you deal with it that makes you the person you are. Maybe I did it all wrong, maybe I should have got help sooner, maybe I should have pushed myself to get out of the relationship (if you can call it that) but as always, it's easier said than done and back then we didn't have all the available help that there is now and who would want to listen to my story? who could stop me thinking and feeling what I did, but just by talking to someone for half an hour and the right professional was a start for me.

BLACK HOLE

People say "hey snap out of it, what's wrong with you"
I'm fighting my own demons every day... if only you knew

Very few days are good, the rest are bad
Someone tell me why I always feel so sad,

I'm clawing my way to get through each day,
And that's how I feel, no matter what you say,

If I could help it I really would,
But this illness is so misunderstood,

Simple things are such a struggle,
My head is constantly in a muddle,

I'm over thinking every tiny thing,
And the rest... well, where to begin,

It's something only yourself will know,
And I hope you never feel this low.

BLACK HOLE EXPLANATION

Well, I finally got out of my constant hell, I moved to a different town which to me felt like a million miles away from everything and everyone I had known for the last 8 years, yep 8 whole years I was in my circle of hell.

The place I moved to was only a bus ride away and change for me was hard... really hard.

Well at least my two children and I had another fresh start, I just hoped I could be strong enough to get through all this and carry on.

Some days I would walk up the high street and feel like I wasn't even in my own body, I felt like a ghost of a person, not sure if that's what 'he' had done to me but I was feeling down, really down.

I would bump into people I knew and had to explain why I had a face like a slapped arse and I would be told to 'snap out of it' and be thankful me and my kids were free at last, of course I was thankful that my kids were safe now (and me), but there was something deeper going on inside me but I just couldn't explain it.

I didn't really have any 'good' days for a long time, the days I classed as good were the ones where I forced a smile for a matter of seconds, the only way I can describe how I felt was that someone gave me a jigsaw puzzle that had been completed then threw it inside my head, so all the pieces were mixed, some pieces were next to each other that just didn't fit and some were scattered everywhere and some parts were even lost.

I didn't want to feel like this and there's nothing anyone could do or say to make it better.

It was like a massive big black heavy cloud looming over me slowly pushing down on me and I was sinking beneath it, into a big black hole... if only that hole would just swallow me up.

I knew I had depression around two years after having my first child but this feeling was something entirely different, the feelings were much stronger and impulsive.

I really wanted people around me because I didn't like being on my own but I also didn't want to face people because when I did it was tiring to smile and pretend. I felt like I was a ghost standing there staring at myself and pretending I was someone I wasn't.

NANNY BET

Well, my beautiful Nan what can I say,
God needed you so he took you away,

No one was ready to let your beautiful soul go,
And we all love you more than you'll ever know,

I wish I came to see you more and for that I regret,
But no one on this earth could come close to you, Nanny 'Bet',

The sky has gained a beautiful star,
And we will see you no matter how far,

Lucky heaven because they have gained you,
But we aren't so lucky because we lost you,

It's a horrible pain that will never go away,
I just want to hold you and for you to stay,

I love you Nan more than I've ever expressed,
And till I see your beautiful face, I'll let you rest,

Goodnight Nan

NANNY BET EXPLANATION

My beautiful kind hearted nan, well she was amazing, had the loveliest smile, the kindest soul and another great cook. No one could make cheese twists; Yorkshire puddings or amazing cakes like her. She used to make all my birthday cakes, one in particular was a jack and jill cake, the detail was beautiful, she always had time to cook and she enjoyed every minute of it, her smile made everyone feel right at home.

When she died, I was already in a bad place mentally and although I worked in the same building as a carer where my Nan lived, (I know I'm an awful person), I didn't go and see her as much as I should have, this was because all day I was wearing my mask and trying to hide the pain that I was mentally going through, I needed to get my day done and get out of there, go home and shut myself away in the dark. My job as a carer didn't last very long because of my constant depression, anxiety and constant mood swings which at this point I didn't understand.

I was feeling like this daily and it really was an emotional roller coaster for me, I felt like I was constantly battling not only myself but the world too.

There were times I did go and say hello to my Nan and Grandad and I remember sitting there thinking I need to cry; I want her to cuddle me and help me and tell me everything was going to be ok but I thought that would have been so selfish of me to put that worry and my problems on her, so my visits were always cut short because I needed to go home and cry, I was always crying at this point, I still didn't know who I was or what my place or purpose was in this world, (to this day I sometimes feel like I still don't know) although its only for short periods of time now and I know I will never see the world as 'normal people' do but I try as best I can.

The medication that I'm on now I will have to take for the rest of life, it helps me so much.

If you feel like you don't know where your place in this world is and your feelings are so overwhelming then please ask for help.

I went into an even deeper downward spiral when I got the dreaded phone call that my nan had gone, that's when I started self-harming, I thought I deserved to be punished for not being a good granddaughter and not seeing her as much as I should have.

The self-harming was happening daily, I felt like I needed to punish myself. I know this might sound strange to some people but I also know that some people will totally relate to this.

RELEASE THE PAIN

I get mad and angry and want to cause myself pain,
So, I get out the knife and cut above my vein,

It's a release that only I understand,
Take it off me and just grab my hand,

I need to be held and let out a tear,
But I'll do it again and that's my fear,

Cut and cut 'til I start to bleed,
Just want to stop it, is all I need,

I hurt inside so I punish myself,
I just want to control this mental health,

After it's done, I feel nothing but shame,
But it's only me I have to blame,

Feel like I've failed every time I cut,
But it's me not you that's stuck in this rut,

I'm sorry I do this and hurt people I love,
Wish someone was looking down from above,

Please make me stop or take away my pain,
Because I can't promise you, I won't do it again,

Cut and cut 'til I start to bleed,
Someone help me is all I plead.

RELEASE THE PAIN EXPLANATION

When my Nan died, I hit an even darker place that I didn't think even existed, I thought I was already at that place and trying to work my way back up, but nope this was darker.

I felt so guilty that I didn't see my Nan as often as I should have. I cried so much one night and was so angry at myself and felt like I needed to punish myself that I didn't even really think about it, I just pulled a knife from the draw and started slicing across my wrist back and forth, back and forth, I was looking at what I was doing, I just knew I needed to harm myself

to make myself feel better. I could feel my wrists start to burn then dropped the knife and pulled my tablets out of the cupboard, I starting swallowing them, one after another until there was none left and I slumped to the floor.

Luckily once they had kicked in, I was sick so most of the tablets came back up, I didn't feel lucky though, I thought I couldn't even kill myself properly, I wouldn't have got any help even if I wasn't sick, I felt like I didn't deserve to be here anyway.

None of my kids were there, (maybe I wouldn't have got to that point if they were). Some people say how could you do that to your poor kids and try and leave them without a mum, but at that point I genuinely thought my kids would have a better life without me, I mean, what mother who doesn't want to be alive deserves her beautiful kids anyway?

I had already put them through so much, seeing all the domestic abuse and what that had done to me physically and mentally, so what was the point anymore, my mind was exhausted.

I didn't sleep well that night, I just grabbed my hair in my hands as hard as I could, like this was going to take away all the bad thoughts and feelings that were going through my head.

I felt dirty, ashamed, sad, angry, but most of all I felt empty inside, like I had been fighting for too long in life and had run out of every ounce of energy I had, I didn't deserve energy, I just wanted to lay there, which I did most of the day, with the TV on but I couldn't hear a word anyone was saying on it, I was just looking straight through them in a daze.

I was an empty shell of a person, just like I was years ago, but this time in a different way.

I had let everyone down and become a selfish person. My dad, my grandad, my family, they were all grieving, so why couldn't I just grieve in a normal way? what made me so different? was my past coming back to bite me in the arse or did I just handle bad situations in a selfish way?

Just needed someone to hold me and tell me everything was going to be OK and that I'm not selfish for doing what I did, but most importantly understand why I did it but I'm my own worst enemy and no one understood me and what was going on in my head, not even I did anymore.

FIVE DAYS

It's been 5 days now and I just want to die,
To say I want to be here would just be a lie,

I'm planning how and planning when,
At least I'll get to see you again,

My babies don't need me I'm just a psycho mum,
Give it time and that will be me done,

You all carry on with your normal lives,
While I sit here staring at the knives,

It's gone deeper than cutting my stupid arm,
Just need someone to keep me from harm,

But there is no one, I'm all alone,
Just want to be somewhere I feel at home,

That place is not hear anymore,
You're all so sick of me I'm just a bore,

I'm constantly tired and can't seem to smile,
But you only have to put up with me for a little while,

I'm saying goodbye in my own little way,
Because I just can't do this every single day,

I feel like I'm suffocating every day,
I know in the end you'll be glad I'm away,

I'm doing this for my babies and of course you,
because I really don't know what I'm going to do,

I can't trust or love not anymore,
And I'm sick of crying on this dirty floor,

I just need to be free from this constant hell,
I'm looking at me and I'll never be well,

I'm sorry my illness made me evil and bad,
And I'm sorry that everyone thinks I'm mad,

But I'm suffocating here and need to go,
I've never ever felt this low,

I love you all so much but life will just go on,
But I'm hurting and tired and I just can't hold on.

FIVE DAYS EXPLANATION

These 5 days were probably the most suicidal i have ever felt (hence the poem) I really did at the time think that everyone who I ever cared and loved about would be better off without me.

I felt that mentally I couldn't carry on, my head was so tired from constantly battling against myself and the demons I was facing every single day. I would lay on my bed everyday thinking about how I would say my final goodbyes to the people I loved, I didn't know where to start, apart from keep telling them that I loved them because I couldn't put my feelings into words.

In my head at that time, I really believed I was worthless and useless to everyone around me and I just wanted to fall asleep and never wake up. I was exhausted from myself and my thoughts and they were just consuming my head.

The overwhelming feeling of needing to go to sleep and not wake up was far greater than having the energy to carry on through another day.

I wasn't diagnosed at this point with my EUPD so I couldn't make sense of my life or what was wrong with me. I know all this sounds strange to some people and believe me it didn't make sense to me either.

I'm in a good place now though and i often sit back and think about my demons and thoughts that nearly cost me my life. I couldn't tell you what stopped me taking my own life because some of them memories are a blur. Obviously, my kids were a big part of my recovery and stopped me on occasions doing something drastic, whenever I thought about them, I thought how could I leave them without a mummy.

But on the other hand, like I said, I couldn't even kill myself properly (so glad I couldn't now).

I remember crying constantly on my kitchen floor just looking at the knives on my kitchen side wondering how I could make it as painless as possible; the overdosing was the best possibility for me but I learnt from the past that I couldn't even do this right which made me feel even more useless, I felt like I was stuck in a cycle that was all to familiar to me. My go I wanted out of that cycle but just didn't know how. I always thought that this was my life forever and nothing was going to change, but believe me when people say that time is a healer (and the right help and medication) I didn't just go to the doctors get put on medication and I was ok, I have been through nearly every antidepressant there is and none of them worked (For me).

I've had family members ringing the crisis line because no one knew what to do with me, I have seen psychiatrists and was even going to section myself, I was literally ripping my hair out, punching my own face, headbutting things, self-harming, suicidal thoughts, compulsive

behaviour, wanting to crash my car into a brick wall, dark thoughts, no sense of belonging, feeling like no one in the world understood me but here I am writing this in the hope that if just one person has these thoughts or feelings, they will seek help or read these poems and explanations and know that someone else does feel and think similar or maybe the same thoughts you're going through, but I'm proof that things can get better and I hope you find your light at the end of your dark tunnel.

YOU

You were the one that caught me when I fell,
You were the one that took me out of my hell,

You made me see that not all men are the same,
You made me feel like I was myself again,

You love me for my flaws and my mental health,
You made me see that actual love is wealth,

You are the one that wipes my river or tears,
You are the one that listens to my fears,

You are always there right by my side,
You're always there with arms open so wide,

You make me laugh every single day,
You always know the right things to say,

You've completed my life and give me hope,
You take the strain when you know I can't cope,

You love me for me and that's all I ask,
You even know when I'm wearing my mask,

You bring me happy when I'm feeling sad,
You bring me laughter when I'm being mad,

You're everything to me an even more,
Thank you for accepting my life before.

Thank you for saving me from total disaster
And showing me that life can be filled with laughter.

YOU EXPLANATION

This is the man that saved me and became my best friend and husband. Without him I don't know where I would be. He brings so much happiness and stability to my life that I couldn't imagine living without him.

He understands and accepts my mental health as this will always be a part of me forever now.

He brings so much laughter to my life which is the best feeling, knowing you can be your crazy self without being judged.

He makes me feel like I belong in this world and I'm not this totally mental human that nobody can love (just like I was told for years before) he is my best friend and we do everything together.

We both didn't have the best start when we got together as we had both been through similar situations but this made us stronger because we knew how we both wanted to be treated and loved and we gave that to each other.

It's not always been easy because of my mental health and there are days or even weeks that I'm not me, but he accepts that, which I will be forever grateful for, no one has shown me the love that this man has and I know that I've got to a place in my life where I am happy and understand where I'm at.

Instead of dreading waking up and feeling like I can't carry on another day, he's there pulling me through. I feel amazed some days when I think back at all the things that have happened and been said to me because from being constantly abused physically and mentally, all the bruises, cuts, marks, and the 'fat slag' this and 'nobody will ever love you', 'you're just nothing in this world', 'you're the ugliest person that i have ever laid eyes on' to then being with someone that is the total opposite. He has never physically or mentally hurt me.

I feel like someone else watching all these good things happen, like it's not happening to me because I don't deserve it.

I was a shell of myself for so long I didn't even know who I was or who I was meant to be, but now I know that I'm a mum that wants to live for her kids and I'm a wife that wants to experience as much as I can in this world with my husband and family but most important.

I'm me again, I'm not perfect I'm far from it, I've made mistakes (huge ones) but I believe everything bad that happens leads you to somewhere good in life.

If what happened to me didn't happen, I wouldn't be writing this now and sharing my own personal story trying to get women/men out of their violent relationships, (physically or mentally,) I wouldn't have met my husband and found myself again, I wouldn't have got the help I wanted/needed, I wouldn't have the beautiful home life I have now and most of all I wouldn't be the best mum I could be. All thanks to 'YOU' my husband, and of course my kids, they have been so patient and understanding I thank them all.

This is the man that saved me and without him I don't know where I would be. He brings so much happiness and stability to my life that I couldn't imagine living without him.

SORRY BABIES

Sorry to my kids, especially my girl,
You shouldn't have had to go through your mum's own hell,

But you two were the people that kept me going,
you and your brother without even knowing,

Your little smiles an innocent love,
Were pure as feathers from a soft white dove,

You wiped my tears an held me tight,
Whenever you saw yet another fight,

I did try to keep you both from any harm,
And tried my hardest to keep things calm,

But you always knew when Mummy had pain,
And I promised you would never see that again,

But again, and again you always did,
By taking your brother and you both hid,

I'm sorry for the things you had to see,
Wish it didn't happen and he just left me be,

I'm sorry you struggle with how life is,
You seeing none of it would be my only wish,

But you and your brother kept alive,
So, anything bad I know you'll survive,

You were both my reason for breathing every day,
But you'll never believe me no matter what I say,

I love you both with every beat of my heart,
And I'm sorry I let a 'man' tear us apart.

Love you both forever

SORRY BABIES EXPLANATION

This is the hardest explanation I have had to write in here because it breaks my heart knowing what my two eldest kids saw, especially my oldest as she was at an age that she understood what was happening around her.

I've sat here for a while thinking of the right words to say but there isn't a different way of saying how sorry I am, there isn't a time machine that would make me go back and change it all for them.

I wanted them to have the chance of being 'typical kids' not fearing what the next day would bring, not wanting to go to school because they were worried about their mummy or frightened and scared that their daddy was going to hit their mummy again and wanting to stop it even though they were so young.

This made it really hard because when your being physically hurt and your child tries to get In the way you retaliate with all your strength to keep your kids safe so if that meant hitting back then that's what I would do but some people think I shouldn't of, but what is the right thing to do, lay there and let your kids see what their daddy was going to do to their mummy or try and help yourself and your kids?...

Most of it was a blur but some things will stick with me forever, like the time I had my son in my arms, he was about 2 and me and 'him' had just got some wardrobes which were in the front room ready to be put together and yet another argument broke out which resulted in me being so hard in the face I fell back against the wardrobes then onto the floor but with my little boy in my arms.

I clung to my baby with all my strength just so he stayed safely in my arms, then I realised if his daddy had missed my face and caught our baby then my baby wouldn't have survived that punch.

My babies would tell me not to let daddy back in the house when he decided to leave but they didn't understand the consequences of what would happen to me/us if I did, we would be in more danger because he would come back angrier looking for revenge for locking the door and not opening it when he TOLD me to.

He would smash the small windows in the front door to get in, or lurk about outside shouting and swearing so again I was trapped, no matter what I did. I couldn't keep my babies safe and as a parent this was the most heart-breaking thing, all you want for your children is for them to be safe and happy and I couldn't give them either.

When your child is wiping your tears and stroking your hair because lumps have been pulled out, your heart literally breaks there and then, which then makes the tears come harder and faster and the guilt and shame consumed me all in that moment sitting on the toilet seat while your child is saying 'its ok mummy, don't worry I'm here' My heart broke and ached for them.

My kids don't know this, (no one did until now), but I was even considering putting them into care just to keep them safe and that was another heart-breaking moment for me because I didn't want to take away their mummy but I wanted to keep them safe and I don't know if I was selfish to carry on letting my kids see the abuse, until i could escape or if keeping them with me they didn't lose the one constant in their life…

I tried so hard to deal with the mental and physical abuse plus me fighting my own mental health and demons and trying to keep my kids safe that I was literally a nervous confused wreck, I always thought that I didn't deserve my kids (sometimes I still do) because the eldest sometimes believes she don't matter to anyone and sometimes feels like she doesn't want to be here and I know that's my fault and I have to live with that forever just like my mental health.

I'm so sorry to them for everything they have seen and how that has impacted on their lives now, I just hope they know that all through the worst times that happened they were the ones that kept me alive.

I love you both so much (and my other two) but the two eldest who were with me on my darkest journey, who kept me in this world today I have no other words apart from sorry and I hope I'm making you proud now.

I'M SORRY

I'm sorry right now that I'm such a bloody mess,
But I'm feeling really down (If you can't already guess),

I feel so overwhelmed with everything I feel,
I just wish so bad there was a magic pill,

I feel lonely and scared, but most of all sad,
I just want to go back to the happy times we had,

Some days I feel like I let everyone down,
And my smiles have disappeared and I'm left with a frown,

I'm sorry I'm so down every single day,
But it won't go away no matter what you say.

I'M SORRY EXPLANATION

When I first met my husband, I couldn't believe that someone finally loved me for me and all my flaws and 'baggage' as 'the ex' called our kids.

'No one will love me with children and take them on as their own,' I was 'damaged goods' and that's how I felt for many years, that I wasn't worthy of anyone's time or love because I was just 'nothing' for so long.

That all changed when I met my soul mate and he became my happy place. he made laugh and still does every day.

First few weeks were amazing with him but then the words and the thoughts and feelings of me not being good enough all came back to haunt me, and what do you do when things like this happen?

You step back, you put up your brick wall, you stop trusting anyone and become the shell of the person that you've always felt you was AGAIN.

I was stood looking at this man that was making me laugh, giving me no reason to doubt him, being gentle and kind but there were the words 'no one will love you ever again, your ugly, you don't deserve to be loved' where whizzing around my head again and again and that's all it took to take me right back to where I didn't want to be. I once again became very depressed very quickly, it was exhausting. Could I ever move on and get past the mental abuse?

The physical abuse was so much easier to get over because black eyes fade, bruises go, foot marks on your skin disappear but words are there. the most powerful and for some people soul destroying. they don't fade away, they don't disappear (for me anyway) they have stayed with me forever and instead of becoming the better person and deal with the mental abuse I let it swallow me up into that dark hole I fought so hard to crawl out of. This wasn't fair on my husband; it wasn't his battle to fight it was mine and I knew I wasn't fighting it well.

Surely this man is too good to be true, surely, he will hurt me, think I'm ugly too, think I don't deserve to be loved so what did I do? I pushed him away, and for that I felt guilty.

Every single day since I first met him, he has called me beautiful, obviously I have never ever felt beautiful because I have had so many years of being called the opposite but it still makes me smile that he thinks that about me.

He just didn't understand me and I couldn't make him understand because only I knew what was whizzing around in my head. I didn't mean to be sad all the time, I didn't mean to push him away and I didn't mean to let my past win, but mental abuse made me feel like he would walk away from me at any time so I better not get too attached.

My EUPD certainly played a part in my thinking process. I couldn't have a stable relationship with the only person I craved to be with, and to this day I think that it will all come crashing down on me and I'm left alone and he won't love me anymore and that's something that I will probably have to live with forever, well I know I will live with it forever.

It made me so sad and feel so guilty that he was now carrying my past with me and I feel like it's not because he wants to but because he has to. I wanted him by my side but I still felt alone because one thing he couldn't carry was my thoughts and these were the most damaging to me I so wanted to smile and be happy with him but my brain just wouldn't let me, it was so hard and I know it was hard for him to watch me fall apart some days into a hole he couldn't get me out of and for that I will always be sorry for, he didn't have to try and understand me, he didn't have to wipe my tears away or listen to what I was trying to tell him but he did and without him I would still be in that hole trying to claw my way out.

He doesn't understand what he has done for me and how he has changed my life and I will forever be thankful to him for that.

TIRED

I wake from 8 hours sleep and I'm tired,
I don't want to get out of bed and begin the day, because I'm tired,

I 'HAVE' to get up and look after the kids, but I'm tired,
I struggle through each day, willing bedtime to hurry up, because I'm tired,

I want to go out with the kids and have lots of fun, but I'm tired,
I want to go out for the day, but planning it is tiring,

I want to do lots of things in life, but I'm just so tired,
My brain is tired, it's tired of fighting myself each an everyday,

It's tired of over thinking all the bad things that might NEVER happen,
It's tired of juggling all these different thoughts and emotions,

It's tired of repeating the same thought process every day,
It's tired of trying just to end up failing, its tired of going two steps forward and 100 back,

It's tired of feeling like you're getting nowhere in life, it's just draining all the time, All the little things to others are massive to me, because I'm so tired. Just wish my mind didn't make me so tired :(

TIRED EXPLANATION

I'm always so tired.

Before my doctor prescribed me with sleeping tablets my brain literally wouldn't switch off, I thought about everything and anything. I thought about scenarios that were beyond my minds control, extreme thoughts like someone shooting or stabbing my children and yes this might sound absolutely crazy to some of you but I'm sure this was related to the abuse I got, and how scared I was of my children getting hurt but the extreme thoughts going round and round in my head would make me so so tired.

I didn't want to get up every morning and open the curtains or see daylight but I had no choice and then out came my mask, the smiling for everyone else around me because if I didn't, I felt like they would read my face and could see the dark thoughts that were constantly going round in my mind, it was exhausting every single day. Some weekends when I didn't have the children, I would lay in bed with the curtains closed and cry and 'think' AGAIN.

My mind was in overdrive and I didn't know how to stop it.

It wouldn't get better and I didn't know why, it wasn't until years later that I was diagnosed with my personality disorder and may have even have PTSD as well as the EUPD due to my past.

It may seem small to what some people have gone through but this is just a little bit of my story, the bits I can manage to write and share with you all. To tell you things that have happened to me which still affect me to this day.

My husband could point to something and even now my natural reaction will sometimes be to flinch. Sometimes I think he's going to work and not coming back because of how unstable I can be.

Not being able to form relationships is a part of this horrible illness. The one thing we can't control is the thoughts and feelings that we all experience in life and that can be tiring in itself, we don't need to have an illness for that but I felt like the only person in the world that was feeling like this, it is such a lonely illness because you think nobody will ever understand what's going on in your head but there are health professionals out there that DO understand and can help.

GREY

Well... I got through the darkness and found the light,
I saw the grey between the black and the white,

I still have days that I mask my smile,
And this could go on for a little while,

But I look back and see just how far I've come,
Mostly that's down to finding 'the one',

When you have bad days just think of the hell,
And the dark days that you knew you wasn't too well,

If you got through them days then you can do it again,
You WILL find a way you just don't know when,

This mental health journey is yours not mine,
Things do change it just takes time,

You may feel alone and like no one will care,
You may do things bad and that's a scare,

But its ok now not to be ok
and I'm sure in time you'll find your own way.

GREY EXPLANATION

Well, what can I say… never thought I would/could get through the darkest times of my life but I did, don't get me wrong I still go through really bad periods in my life but don't we all.

I've just learnt to cope with them better because of professional intervention and the right medications.

I got through that dark dark tunnel I never thought would end and here I am today writing about some of my life experiences through poems, because that was how I always tried to deal with the lowest feelings and times of my life.

With writing, it's me that understands it, all my crazy thoughts and messed up head just trying to work out who I was and where I was going in life, and nobody can take away what you think, feel and write, it's yours and yours only and a great way to try and understand yourself and also look back at your life through your writing.

I did it myself and still think, my god that was my life, whether it's a short period of time or a long period of time, just knowing I got through it was the biggest achievement for me, and if I can help one person get out of their dark place they are in then this was all worth my time, tears and sharing my poems with you.

It was very hard sharing what I have kept to myself for so many years, but it's out there now and I know some people might not like this or judge me or think these poems are crap or boring but it's MY story and I just wanted to help some people and let them know that they are not alone in what they think or feel because I have been there, been through the mental abuse, physical abuse, self-harming, all sorts of medications, lots of health professionals, feeling alone, being alone, suicidal thoughts and much more, but I hope my story will help guide you through your dark tunnel.

People may think 'well I've been through worse than what you have' but abuse is abuse no matter how big or small, it still has the same effect on women/men's mental state of mind which in turn could have the same result in mental health issues or not being able to have form stable relationships, trust issues and lots more. It affects people in different ways and I feel I have had the worst thoughts and feelings only people at rock bottom could possibly understand.

I hope you enjoyed reading just a small part of my life that I've shared with you all.

MY LIFE NOW

My life right now has gone from strength to strength, don't get me wrong I still have days where I don't want to talk to anyone, I feel exhausted when I've not done anything or I can't snap out of my blackness and I still use my mask but for me that is still my safe place, at least then there are no questions asked about your feelings that you really don't want to answer.

My partner is the only person that always knows how I'm feeling (even with my mask) but he always knows the right thing to do weather that's leaving me be or making me smile or taking the strain from me, he will sometimes do the kids dinner or baths and I'm so grateful to him for them small things which at the time seem like big jobs to me.

He still carries on loving me through all of this but like he said, my mental health is a part of me and that's what makes me myself and he loves me for it…

Keep going and do things that are out of your comfort zone, it could open up a world of opportunities without you even realising it, you will start to feel stronger and better. Some weeks the bad days will outweigh the good but doesn't mean your failing it means you're trying and to someone with mental health issues that is the biggest step 'trying'.

We all want them bad days to become fewer and start living and laughing but one step at a time.

During my worst times I spent so long in my bed with the curtains shut, crying or sleeping that now I make it a rule for myself and my daughter that when you're in your bad place, get up and open them curtains and do something, just one thing, fold the washing, clean a cupboard just do something, but with them curtains open, might not work for you but it does for me and my daughter.

Someone one day will understand and love you the way you deserve.

You can't escape mental health but you can learn to cope and live with it.

Hopefully someone WILL love you for you and your mental health because that will always be a part of who you are no matter how big or small.

www.ingramcontent.com/pod-product-compliance
Lightning Source LLC
Chambersburg PA
CBHW070801220526
45467CB00017B/723